Autophagy

Find Out How Autophagy Can Make You Lose Weight Fast. How To Reduce Inflammation And Activate The Anti-Aging Process, With The Help Of The Ketogenic Diet And Intermittent Fasting

By: Serena Stephens

considered both accurate and truthful when it comes to the recounting of facts. As such, any use, correct or incorrect, of the provided information will render the Publisher free of responsibility as to the actions taken outside of their direct purview. Regardless, there are zero scenarios where the original author or the Publisher can be deemed liable in any fashion for any damages or hardships that may result from any of the information discussed herein.

Additionally, the information in the following pages is intended only for informational purposes and should thus be thought of as universal. As befitting its nature, it is presented without assurance regarding its prolonged validity or interim quality. Trademarks that are mentioned are done without written consent and can in no way be considered an endorsement from the trademark holder.

Table of Content

Introduction

Thank you so much for downloading the book *autophagy: find out how fasting improves your health. An indispensable guide that helps you heal your body and lose weight with the self-cleaning autophagy system.* In this book will talk about autophagy and how to achieve true autophagy from various diets. Many people don't know this, but this method has known to help people achieve youth and better health overall.

 If you're someone looking to meet overall health benefits, whether it be in the gym or outside the gym or if you want to feel younger then make sure you start following the information provided to you and use it because it will help you achieve that goal. Believe it or not, many people believe that this process will help you tremendously to not only put on muscle but to feel healthy overall, and many scientists have proved it. Keeping that in mind there's no way for you to go but to achieve autophagy if your goal is to put on muscle and to lose fat at the same time.

Moreover, this diet will help you to achieve proper health and well-being. With that being said, I hope you enjoy this book as we have genuinely handcrafted the information here for you to achieve optimal health and success. Most importantly, make sure that you enhance your diet and eating habits in the long term for you to see progress. Don't worry and we will be talking about that as well later on in this book.

Chapter 1: Autophagy 101

You might be wondering what Autophagy is, and this chapter will clarify that and help you understand what Autophagy is and how to follow it the right way later on in this chapter. One thing you have to realize with Autophagy is that it has a cell rejuvenation process, which allows you to get rid of the old cells and therefore, will enable you to build new cells. What Autophagy does is allow you to get the cell to survive stress from external environments. Moreover, it allows you to withstand internal pressure. When it comes to achieving youth and better appearance, there is no better way to go about it then to follow Autophagy or to achieve true Autophagy through diet. There are many stages to Autophagy, which is what we're going to talk about in this chapter, so you have a clear idea of what the stages are.

You might have heard claims such as Autophagy having anti-aging properties, and there is some truth behind it. When you are following an eating protocol related to fasting, your body will start a process known as Autophagy. Autophagy is a process when your cells primarily eat themselves and produce newer and stronger ones this process is known as Autophagy. When you are regularly eating, your body has to work hard on digesting the foods which you are consuming and then doesn't have the time or energy to activate Autophagy. Which is why you will see amazing results when Autophagy because when you are fasting, you are not digesting any food hence having more time for your body to activate the process of rejuvenating new cells. For you to see amazing results from Autophagy, you will have to fast for at least 12 to 16 hours. The reason being is that your body will have burned out all the glycogen in your liver to get the process started, another thing to remember is to not fast for two days at a time, as this is when Autophagy slowly drops. Overall if your goal is to live longer, you need to have an autophagy process running in a healthy manner which fasting provides you. However, Autophagy could also be achieved thru a Ketogenic diet. Even though it isn't ideal, it is still possible for you to obtain true Autophagy from a Ketogenic diet. The main criteria behind it would be for you to ensure that you are getting enough breaks between foods so that your body can start the process of Autophagy. Keep in mind there are stages before you reach Autophagy.

The first one is induction, then comes the assembly and for-mation of autophagosomes, third comes the docking and fusion with lysosomal membranes and finally occurs degradation. Mostly how it works is first, your body will have everything to recover and digest. Once it has understood that it has done everything you can, it will now take the cells to start breaking them down and building up new ones slowly. Apple specifically targets cells which are dying or degrading and fill them up with new ones. Our body is brilliant when it comes to which cell to recover and which they shouldn't recover. Which is why Autophagy is such a quick process that the body does, it will only fix the cells that need to be fixed. Most of the time, especially beginners, the body will break down most of the cell's since most of the cells have not been broken down or been recycled. It is essentially your body recovering new batteries to make sure that you stay healthy for an extended period, and they don't get old.

The benefits of Autophagy and heart

As you might know, heart disease is one of the biggest killers when it comes to conditions. Autophagy has shown to reduce the risk of heart diseases; the way it works is pretty simple. Autophagy has reduced the levels of LDL, which leads to heart attacks. Autophagy has also shown to lower blood pressure levels, and high blood pressure is also one of the many reasons why people tend to have heart complications.

There are many other fitness experts and professional doctors claiming that Autophagy works to reduce the risk of heart diseases. Even though there have been showing studies to back these claims up, they were done on animals. To confirm these claims, we need to make sure that these studies have been backed up on human studies.

Nonetheless, there is still some considerable evidence to follow Autophagy if your goal was to reduce the risk of heart diseases. One way Autophagy can help you to reduce the risk of heart disease is by lowering the amount of sugar present in your bloodstream, and this has shown to decrease the risk of heart diseases in humans. Making it a plus point of Autophagy, so if you are looking to lower the risk of heart diseases the best way possible without following any diets, then Autophagy is the answer for you. But make sure you consult with your physician before you start any plan.

Autophagy and insulin

Autophagy plays a massive role in how your insulin production. When you are eating foods, your insulin tends to spike up and down, resulting in more frequent insulin spikes. This is where Autophagy comes into play, what Autophagy does is that it keeps your insulin stable, therefore keeping your insulin stable throughout the day. More specifically, Autophagy keeps your insulin from not spiking up at all, which will help you become more insulin sensitive.

You must have insulin sensitivity as it will help you reduce the risk of diabetes and many other diseases related to having higher levels of insulin. But the best thing that comes with having a more significant level of insulin sensitivity would be the fact that you digest food a lot better. The more insulin sensitive you are, the better chances of you absorbing the food and converting it into energy would be, as compared to when you are not so insulin sensitive you will most likely store it into your fat reserves. With that said, you must have better insulin sensitivity for overall health.

Autophagy affects your insulin in a very positive way, so make sure that you are using this tool, as it will increase insulin sensitivity in your body. Make sure that you give Autophagy a try, as it will help you become more insulin sensitive and also lower the risk of many diseases such as diabetes.

The benefits of Autophagy

As you know, there are plenty of benefits when it comes to Autophagy. There are not only health benefits, but there are also some mental health benefits which might interest you. Let's talk about some of the health benefits related to Autophagy. The main benefit which you will notice once you start following this eating protocol is the ability to lose body fat at a rapid level.

The truth is that many people can lose body fat with the help of Autophagy, and the best thing about it is that you don't have to change your diet don't eat during the fasting window. Another benefit related to Autophagy is the ability to rejuvenate your cells; this process is also known as Autophagy. Meaning that you will slow your aging process, which to me sounds like a benefit I need! Autophagy can also help you detoxify your digestive system.

As you know, you are not eating for an extended period when following an autophagy eating protocol. Therefore you will give your intestine a break and overall help you clean any issues or any problems related to digestion. Thus resulting in better absorption when you do eat, and absorbing all the nutrients provided to the body. Autophagy has been shown to increase mental focus, as there are no studies to back it up it has been noticed by many followers of this eating protocol so you may or may not see it. Overall there are many benefits to Autophagy, and we will talk about them even later on in this book.

How effective is Autophagy

Since you know the benefits to Autophagy, let's talk about how effective Autophagy can be. First of all, if your goal is to lose body fat, then there is no better way to go about it rather than to follow Autophagy. Many experts suggest that Autophagy can be of great use when you are looking to lose weight, and it is not just saying it many users can back up those results. Another that makes Autophagy effective is the ability to be more consistent.

When you have no diet restrictions, it becomes straightforward for users to become more consistent. Once you become more compatible with your diet, the chances of you seeing more results go up tremendously, which is also one of the reasons why Autophagy is a very effective way to lose body fat or achieve health and fitness goals. After you put all of these into consideration, you will notice that Autophagy is one of the most effective methods of losing fat, getting healthier, and staying more consistent with your diet. There is no way around consistently if you want your plan to be more productive, make sure you follow this plan to the tee if you're going to see amazing effective results.

Why you should follow Autophagy

Since you now know the importance of Autophagy, It all boils down to the question of how vital Autophagy is to your health and why you should consider Autophagy. Since we have spoken about the many benefits of Autophagy, it is a no-brainer that Autophagy can help you with a lot of things. Autophagy can help you lose body fat, have better gut health, lower the risk of heart diseases, and lower the risk of diabetes. Which is one of the reasons why you should consider Autophagy, also Autophagy helps you with is the ability to think a lot better.

Once you start Autophagy, your mind will clear up, and therefore you'll be able to think a lot better at your work or anything that you are doing, which involves mental focus. Another reason why you should consider Autophagy is the simple reason because it keeps you more consistent. As we talked about before, consistency is the key to success in anything. The way Autophagy keeps you more consistent is by giving you loads of freedom, which will help you say more logical for a long time. If your goal is to see long-term results, then you need to follow Autophagy, as it will give you all the benefits and also help you stay more consistent.

Chapter 2: Benefits of autophagy

Let us talk about the health benefits in further length. Many people know there are numerous benefits to autophagy; the major ones are weight loss and cell rejuvenation. Even though these are great benefits, there are many more which autophagy provides you with.

In this chapter, we will talk about all the benefits that come along autophagy. There are many compelling benefits which you might not even know about, so we will go step by step thru each interest. If you are iffy about starting autophagy, then this chapter might turn you on to the idea of fasting. Without wasting any more time, let's talk about the positives of autophagy and how it can help you.

Weight-loss in a healthy manner

As you know, there are many ways to lose weight. However, one of the most popular methods being used to lose weight is autophagy, and there is a good reason behind it. Many people don't know this, but autophagy is perhaps the best way for someone to lose "body fat" instead of "bodyweight." When following most diets, followers tend to lose a ton of weight, but most of the time it is muscle and water weight they are losing.

On the other hand, autophagy makes you lose more body fat. Here is how it works, when you are autophagy for a prolonged period, you have burned out all your glycogen stores. Which makes the body hit your reserves, and that of course, is your body fat. You will be burning more body fat, instead of muscle mass or glycogen, which makes it ideal for people looking to lose weight. Also, as you know, autophagy plays a huge role in affecting your hormones. Your insulin will flat line, and your growth hormone will go up, this will prime your body to burn body fat instead and will do so in a healthy manner.

Now the main reason why autophagy works is pretty simple when you break your fast you have a tiny eating window. This allows you to stay in a caloric deficit, which makes you lose weight in the long run. Unless you binge eat, you will healthily lose weight. According to a 2014 study, people following autophagy lost a significant amount of body weight. Autophagy was found to reduce weight by 3-8% over 3-24 weeks. When examined even further, the participants lost 0.55 lbs. a week on average. However, participants who followed the alternative day autophagy lost 1.65 pounds a week, making it a much better-suited tool for people looking to lose weight.

Another way autophagy is healthier when compared to other weight-loss diets is the fact that there are no restrictions on foods. When people follow different diets it makes it very hard for them to follow since they have to eat every two hours and many other jargons, autophagy makes it very simple for you as there isn't a lot to think about. Where different diets make your weight loss goals your job, autophagy makes it super easy for you, and this makes autophagy a healthy and sustainable way to lose bodyweight. Overall, autophagy is a very healthy and sustainable way to lose body-fat. If you are looking to get rid of excess body fat, then you have nothing else to look for, autophagy is the answer for you. Besides weight loss, autophagy comes with other benefits, which we already talked about. However, now we will go into further details of the health benefits autophagy comes with when you start.

Increased longevity

There have been many studies showing that autophagy can boost longevity. As you might know by now that autophagy can help with cell rejuvenation or also known as autophagy, this process enables you to get rid of the old and weak cell and replace it with newer stronger ones. This process has shown to increase longevity and overall well-being, which is one of the reasons why autophagy can help you live a longer life.

Moreover, some studies are showing that reducing calories in animals by 30% to 40% has shown to increase their lifespan. However, there is no study done on humans claiming such. Nonetheless, some studies are suggesting that monkeys that ate less lived longer. However, there was another study indicating that it wasn't the case on 25-year-old long research done by another party.

Although there is no actual study backing these claims up, it does show that people who ate less had a fewer risk of diseases which could lead to longevity. Which is excellent news when looking at it from that angle, there is a lot of disease prevention that comes with autophagy, but we will talk about those later in this chapter? However, the main thing to remember would be the fact that autophagy helps with autophagy, which enables you to rejuvenate cells, which makes it very evident that autophagy can help you with longevity and overall well-being, which is a great thing to consider.

Prevent diseases

There are many diseases present in today's day and age, and it very common to meet someone suffering from one. Which means, we need to figure out a way to reduce the risk of diseases for overall health and well-being? Intermittent has shown to lower risk of many diseases, and we will be discussing all the conditions autophagy can help getting rid. One of the many diseases autophagy could be Alzheimer's and Parkinson's.

As you know, autophagy helps with boost brain health and to lower the risk of neurogenic diseases. Some studies are showing that autophagy can help reduce the risk of depression, even though some people might not consider this a condition; it is still a significant issue in our society. Autophagy has also shown to reduce cholesterol, a 2010 study on overweight women found that autophagy improved hosts of health complications including cholesterol levels(LDL) and blood pressure which is also known as the silent killer.

Autophagy also helps with reducing type 2 diabetes, and there was one study done on men, which showed that autophagy helped them stop insulin treatment. Although we don't recommend, you try this if you have type 2 diabetes that goes to show you the power of autophagy and insulin resistance.

Nonetheless, many studies are suggesting that autophagy can lower the risk of diabetes. Another devastating disease which autophagy helps getting rid of would be heart diseases. As you know, autophagy enables you to get rid of hypertension, which leads to heart issues. Once your blood pressure drops down, your heart will be working a lot more efficiently, allowing you a healthier life.

In regards to a healthier life, autophagy has also shown to reduce the risk of obesity. One study done on obese women suggested that autophagy reduced the risk of obesity in women, which makes sense as it helps you lose and manage body weight. One of the primary diseases which autophagy could help reduce the risk of is cancer, even though it hasn't been proven yet. Many scientists believe autophagy for a prolonged period could help you get rid of cancer.

These facts about autophagy show you how autophagy can help you get free of many diseases, and some have been backed up with detailed studies, whereas others are still being researched.

Nonetheless, you can't say that about other diets out there. Autophagy will help you to get rid of many things, and prevent you from further having any diseases. There is no better way of getting out of illness or problems without the use of modern medicine, and autophagy is so robust that it will also boost your immune system which will help you avoid small issues like the common flu. All in all, there are many rejuvenating properties which come along with autophagy so don't overlook it and keep all the positives in mind before you look at the negatives.

Reduce stress and inflammation

Autophagy has shown a significant reduction in inflammation. As you know, information causes a lot of many chronic diseases such as Alzheimer's, dementia, obesity, diabetes, and much more. Now, there are many ways that autophagy helps you get rid of inflammation. The first one being autophagy, as you know autophagy helps you with cell rejuvenation cleans up itself by eating out the old self and rejuvenating them with the newer stronger ones. If your body does not rejuvenate itself with more new cells, the older ones have stayed for an extended period of time can cause inflammation.

As you know, the average diet does not allow for cell rejuvenation to happen, and this is where autophagy comes in as it has been proven to help with the process of autophagy. Another way autophagy enables you to get rid of inflammation would be by producing ketones. When your autophagy your body uses up all the glycogen stores which makes it start using stored fat for fuel, and when fats are broken down for energy ketones are produced. One of the most popular ketones in your body will block a part of your immune system, which is responsible for inflammatory disorders. Another way autophagy helps you lower the risk of inflammation is by making you insulin sensitive, and when your body becomes insulin resistant, you will be holding much glucose in your bloodstream. More glucose in your blood will create inflammation and autophagy allows your body to get rid of all the glucose, which helps you reduce inflammation in your body.

Now that we've talked about many ways autophagy enables you to reduce inflammation, let's talk about how autophagy can help you get rid of stress. You see inflammation and stress go hand in hand. If you have high levels of inflammation, chances are your stress levels are going to be higher. Which means that if you lower your inflammation, you will reduce your stress levels, and as you know, autophagy helps with better brain function? Autophagy enables you to send better signals to your brain, which would equal a better functioning brain.

When your mind is functioning at its highest peak, your levels of stress dropdown, better brain function will also help you get rid of any stress you might be having, and having overall better health can help you reduce weight. Overall, all the health benefits you get from autophagy will help you get rid of your weight or at least lowly it. Which means, even if you are not facing pressure, autophagy will help you have a better functioning brain and also help you get rid of any mental fog or stress you might be dealing? What that in mind, always make sure you consult a physician if you are noticing much more stress than you can handle, as it can be something severe and not fixable by autophagy.

Body detox and cell cleaned

Detoxing your body is very important when it comes to living a long healthy life, many people detox their body thru juice cleanse or other methods out there when the truth is that they don't work. Time and time again, autophagy has shown to help detox your body in both the cellular level and digestive level, which means autophagy is a lot more superior when it comes to cleaning your body.

As you know, from cellular level autophagy detoxifies your body with the process of autophagy, what this process does it eat out the bad cells and replace it with healthier and much stronger cells. Through this process, you will notice benefits such as a stronger immune system, prevention of diseases, and insulin sensitivity. It has also shown to reduce the risk of cancer, which is a great thing to know. Overall, this is how autophagy detoxifies your body from a cellular level. Let's talk about how autophagy helps you detoxify from a digestive level standpoint.

People say that your gut is your second brain, and studies are showing how your stomach and mind are connected. Which means if your digestive system isn't functioning at its absolute peak, then chances are your brain won't either? It is essential to have a gut which is clean and working correctly, and intermittent helps a lot with this process.

It has been shown that autophagy can help you clean out your gut and intestines out of debris and junk. Sometimes, we must give your digestive system a break from eating all those foods regularly. Once you start your fast your body will begin to slowly get rid of all the toxins present in your gut, you see when you are eating all the time your body doesn't get a chance to clean itself.

Your body has to focus on digesting the food instead of cleaning out the toxins when you give your body a break from eating. It will start to clean out its gut. Which makes this process great for people who are fasting, when you have a high functioning gut, it will help you digest your food a lot better and also think better? The detoxifying body helps you tremendously with lowering the risk of diseases, which will help you live a longer life.

By now, you can see the pattern, and autophagy helps you from every single place to prevent diseases and many other complications. Which means there are more positives than negatives with autophagy, as we go along in this chapter, you will learn more benefits when it comes to autophagy? However, remember that these will only work unless you do; you have to follow autophagy the right way to see these benefits. With that being said, I hope you have learned a lot from this book as we are almost halfway through it! Now let's move on to another benefit.

Improved insulin sensitivity

As you know, autophagy helps you get more insulin sensitive, which allows you with many things. To understand it better, let me explain to you how insulin works. Every time you eat a meal, your insulin spikes up, then insulin is used to shuttle food either to muscle or your fat store.

When you have too much glycogen in your bloodstream, your body will send that energy to your fat stores. Whereas if you're insulin sensitive, your body will send the glycogen to muscle stores and will be used for energy. When you are insulin sensitive, you are more likely to use up all the glycogen from your food faster, and not requiring your glycogen to be converted into fats.

How autophagy helps with curing insulin resistance is by using up all the glycogen stores, making your body use up fat stores and when you eat food again, it will use up all the glycogen and shuttle it straight to the muscle mass to be used for energy instead of being stored into fat. That is how autophagy helps you become more insulin sensitive, the benefits of being insulin sensitive are many. Once you become insulin sensitive, you will notice more mental energy and less mental fog, and you will also see less fat being stored in your body which makes it ideal for people looking to lose fat and or gain muscle.

Being insulin sensitive will also help you gain more muscle since most of the energy will be sent out to your muscle stores. It will be used to build stronger muscles instead of storing it into fat. Being insulin sensitive is a must, as it will also help you get rid of possible diseases such as type 2 diabetes. All in all, autophagy helps you tremendously with insulin sensitively, which will overall help you live a healthier life.

Increased production of neurotrophic growth factor
Believe it or not, autophagy affects your brain in a significant way. It all happens from the help of brain-derived neurotrophic growth factor, also known as (BDNF), this helps promote neuroplasticity. Neuroplasticity is your brain's ability to migrate and shapeshift, and this helps our brain to produce new brain cells. Once you have an ample supply of BDNF, we can preserve older cells while producing new brain cells. Which means your brain will be healthy and will keep growing because of the new

cells coming. Multiple studies are showing that autophagy to improve brain-derived neurotrophic growth factor, more specifically when it has to do with synapses; this is where your neurotransmitter travel cell to cell.

Autophagy has shown to promote this, and there was a study done where it showed autophagy in process for 12 to 16 hours has shown to increase levels of brain-derived neurotrophic growth factor by around 50-400%. Now we know that autophagy helps promote (BDNF), more explicitly, autophagy helps when it comes down to synapses. It improves what is known as synaptic plasticity, and this helps modulate our moods better. For instance, we can strengthen a synapse or weaken a synapse. This process enables you to be in the moment when you need to be happy or scared; this will help you modulate that accordingly.

In layman's term, this process helps us change our mood and be reactive at the moment. For example, if you need to be more focused, you will be able to because you are modulating it. When your brain-derived neurotrophic growth factor increases, so do your (BDNF) expression. This process helps you produce more brain cells and protect more brain cells, and this affects your cells at a genetic level altering our DNA. Which makes autophagy one of the best ways to protect your brain, and this gives your mind all the help it needs to preserve and recycle out old cells.

Another thing which it helps with is producing more growth hormone, and there was a study done where it showed upwards of a 4000% increase in growth hormone levels. Which is huge when it comes to improvements, as you know, growth hormone is responsible for many things of them being weight loss. It is a plus to have higher amounts of growth hormone, in both men and women. I know that the information was very scientific, so to put in straightforward terms, your brain will rejuvenate a lot quicker.

It will also help you with controlling your moods, which will make it easy to adapt at the moment. Brain-derived neurotrophic growth factor will also help you produce higher levels of growth hormone and serotonin, which are both crucial for mental well-being. Overall, this makes autophagy one of the best brain improving eating patterns out there. For readers looking for mental clarity and fewer moods swings throughout the day, autophagy is your answer to all.

Boost immune system

There is a reason why having a healthy immune system is fundamental, as it will help you get less sick and be more "immune" to disease. Autophagy has shown to increase the immune system, so we will talk about how it boosts the immune system. There was a study done on stem cells when it comes down to autophagy, more specifically, they took a look at how the stem cells rejuvenated.

The study concluded that autophagy depleted white blood cells, which is precisely what we want so our body can produce better and more efficient batteries, which lead to more production of stem cells and lesser of white cells. Once you start to get rid of your old white blood cells, you will begin to produce new ones which will overall help you recover faster. This study also found that there was a reduced amount of protein kinase A (PKA), which allows the stem cells to regenerate. If you have a lower amount of (PKA), this means that it will enable the cells to turn on the regeneration mode, which will allow them to create new cells.

As you know, autophagy has shown to reduce insulin levels, which is a great thing for someone looking to boost their immune system. There was a study done showing that high amounts of insulin levels, prevented t cells from doing its job effectively. The t cells are here to suppress inflammation and to fight off illness; t cells are most of the time responsible for getting rid of toxins which cause disease and inflammation. When your insulin levels are high, t cells are not performing at their highest potential, which creates our immune system to the dropdown.

When you are fasting, there isn't a requirement for insulin spikes, which lets our body help the t cells work at a higher level and overall boosting our immune system. Since you aren't eating for a long time, this will give your gut a break. When you eat a big meal, around 70% of the blood and energy goes to your stomach to digest it. Which means when you are autophagy you, give your body a chance to recover. Everything is healing when you are fasting, which includes the digestive system. Meaning, your gut will be working a lot more effectively once you have given it some time to heal.

 As you know, digestion plays a massive role in both our mental health and immune system, about 60% of our immune system is in our colon, which means when you are autophagy, you are recovering your whole body and overall boosting your immune system. You will be doing yourself a tremendous service if you can manage to boost your immune system, and with all the backed up science showing how autophagy can help you promote your immune system and reduce many other health problems, there is no reason not to start autophagy as soon as possible.

More energy and muscle mass increased

Even if your goal isn't to put on more muscle, it is still good to have more muscle mass as it helps you with many things. However, the main thing having higher amounts of muscle mass helps you with would be a fat loss; having a higher muscle mass will help you burn fatter since it increases your metabolic rate. Don't worry and you don't have to look like a bodybuilder for that to happen; nonetheless, it is essential to have the right amount of muscle mass, especially for women.

Autophagy has shown to increase and preserve muscle mass, so let's talk about how that happens. There was a study done between two groups of me one followed a 16/8 autophagy method, and the others followed, whereas the other followed a regular eating pattern. Both groups followed the same workout and the same diet, and just the group autophagy would eat in the eight-hour window. What they noticed after eight weeks was, both the groups gained and preserved the same amount of muscle, but the group who were following the autophagy lost more fat.

This shows that autophagy not only helped followers gain muscle and preserve it, but it also helped them lose fat simultaneously. The main reason behind that is growth hormone, as you know; autophagy has shown to increase growth hormone in our bodies. What growth hormone mainly does, it allows a lot less muscle breakdown and to burn more fat, which is one of the main reasons why autophagy is so beneficial for building and preserving muscle mass.

Another great benefit of autophagy, as you know, is higher energy levels, and there is a reason behind it. Many people know how it feels to have a sugar crash, you feel tired and lethargic, and the culprit behind it is insulin. When insulin is spiked up, your energy level goes down as this gives your brain a signal to relax. When you are autophagy, there are no insulin spikes throughout the day, which provides you with more energy to stuff.

Another reason why you have more energy when you are in autophagy is that your body goes into a fight or flight response and since your body is in a normal starvation mode, it feels like for it to get food it needs to hunt. Which is when your body produces more adrenaline throughout the day, which gives you more energy as you go along? Just be aware, at the beginning of your autophagy journey, you might feel less energized.

The reason behind it is because your body is still getting used to these changes, but after a week or two, you should start to notice more energy. Use the power to get more work done at work and gym. In my opinion, and this is the most significant benefit which comes along with autophagy. More energy makes you feel a lot better when you are looking towards making it thru those long days.

These are all the main benefits which come along when you start fasting, and the benefits genuinely outweigh all the negatives autophagy might come with. These benefits can be life-changing to most people, lowering the risk of diseases and increasing longevity it's a fantastic thing to have. Autophagy provides you with that and then some, with that being said It is now time for you to pick an autophagy plan and start implementing it which is what we are going to talk about in the next chapter.

Chapter 3: Working out and meditation

When following autophagy, one of the main things you need to consider would be diet exercise and rest. In this chapter, we will go into depts on how you can ensure that all of the items listed above are in check. Many of you might be falling back on either three of these aspects, the sooner you realize which one it is and fix it, the better.

Diet and nutrition

In the previous chapter, we already talked about the importance of diet and nutrition. Let's further discuss it to ensure that you are optimizing this aspect as well. Having the right diet and nutrition can either break you or make you in the realm of fitness and health. The simplest way to ensure that your diet and nutrition is on point is to keep it simple, by that I mean not following any crazy diets which will hinder your goals and success.

The ideal to go about it would be to eat healthy foods during your eating window. Please do not make your food intake very complicated, if your goal is to lose weight merely being a little bit of caloric deficit and eat good vegetables and meat will do the trick. This will provide you with optimal nutrition while striving you towards your goals. The reason why we keep bringing up diet and nutrition, Is to show you that you can follow autophagy without overthinking. If your diet or nutrition plan is too complicated for you and becomes a chore, then chances are you're not developing the right strategy. The next time you're planning out your food intake, make sure that this isn't a chore for you and More so of a lifestyle.

How autophagy affects your body

Autophagy works uniquely, so let's talk about it. When you're following an autophagy type of eating protocol, you are going to a starvation mode. When you're into starvation mode, your body thinks that it's not getting enough food and therefore it starts breaking down your fat stores.

The same thing would happen to our ancestors, they would go without food for a couple of days and once they did find food they would eat much food to store it into body fat stores so they can use it later on. We are merely following a diet, which was used by our ancestors. Believe it or not, there are a lot healthier than us, and they didn't have any diseases such as diabetes and so on.

Nonetheless, let's get into the science of intermittent fasting. When you are fasting, your body will burn off all the glycogen and your bloodstreams for a couple of hours. Once it has burnt out all the glycogen in your blood, it will start to use your fat stores for energy. Which is where the magic happens, you will burn more fat throughout the day than you would following any other diet, which makes intermittent fasting, one of the best foods to follow if your main goal is to lose fat or to lower the risk of diseases.

Eating wrong foods can counter those effects

Eating the wrong foods can counter those effects during intermittent fasting. Even though when you're following intermittent fasting, you're allowed to eat whatever you want. However, that doesn't mean it is a most optimal way to go about it, here's the thing if you're going to ensure that you're not countering the effects from autophagy then you need to eat the right foods.

Since you already know the right foods to eat when intermittent fasting, let's talk about the wrong foods that you shouldn't eat when you're following an autophagy type of the protocol. The first thing you should not eat would be anything which would be considered junk food, even though most people have seen success through eating junk food while intermittent fasting. We don't recommend that you do the same, because the chances are you will store that food into fats quickly then you would eating healthy foods. Another reason why you should not eat junk food while intermittent fasting is because it would not help you lower the risk of any diseases. Even though autophagy is a powerful way to reduce the risk of conditions, it can't be countered without the consumption of healthy foods.

On the other hand, eating junk food by itself will increase the risk of heart diseases and diabetes. To keep everything simple, stay away from food, which would be considered fast foods. Once you manage to do that, you will be in a lot better place.

Important food groups for nutrition

There are many essential food groups to consider when following intermittent fasting. To keep things very simple, eat foods which were available thousands of years ago. These include meats, vegetables, and some grains here and there. The idea that you need to consider to eat foods which are low on the glycemic index, so you don't increase your insulin levels when you do eat those foods.

When you spike your insulin level consistently, you put yourself in the risk of attracting type 2 diabetes. Which is why you need to research the types of food you're eating, so make sure whatever you're eating has a low glycemic index. Most of the time, foods such as brown rice, meat, and vegetables tend to have a shallow glycemic index.

Meaning they will not spike your insulin very quickly, and it will take time for you to burn off those calories from the food giving you a sustained amount of energy throughout the day. This is where you want to be when following intermittent fasting, and you need to have a sustained amount of energy throughout the day.

The main three food groups of nutrition would be carbohydrates protein and fats. It would be best if you made sure that all three of these are coming from good healthy food. It would help if you were careful more on the carbohydrates side of the nutrition, as are many carbohydrates which will spike your insulin very quickly. Eat carbs, which are low on the glycemic index, and you will be fine.

Do autophagy and exercise go together?

Many people feel that autophagy exercise does not go together, just because you're starving yourself throughout the day. However, the truth is when following an autophagy type of the protocol, you have terrific workouts, and there's a reason behind it.

When you're autophagy, your body goes into starvation mode when your body is in the starvation mode, and it raises your adrenaline, which is why some people notice better mental focus while fasting. When your adrenaline goes up, you will have more energy to do physical tasks because your body feels like it needs to be fighting for food, which is why you will have a lot of energy throughout the day especially when you going to work out. From personal experience, I can tell you that I've had one of my the best workouts while following autophagy and that too while I was in the fast. The best part about working out while intermittent fasting is that you will burn fat for energy instead of glycogen for power.

It is meaning that you will gain more fat loss benefits from working out while intermittent fasting. Some have said that autophagy lowers their strength levels, but it is not noticeable if you're not a powerlifter. If your goal is merely to lose weight that autophagy is a great idea to be falling while working out.

Go for high-intensity workouts after eating

Here is the truth, the best way to burn fat when falling autophagy is to follow a high-intensity type of workout plan. When you follow a high-intensity kind of workout plan, you'll consume a lot more calories for an extended period. Ideally should be working out right after you have broken your fast, this will put you in a position where you have some food in you to burn off. High-intensity workouts work great if your goal is to have better cardiovascular health and to burn off some fat.

Ideally should be doing a cardio workout, at least three to four times a week to ensure that your fat is melting off but in conjunction of that, you need to make sure that your workouts are high intensity. As this will not only burn off more fat, but it will raise your hormones, which will help you live a better life or healthier life, I should say. The next time you're planning out your workouts, make sure that they are high intensity and short. This will ensure that you are getting closer to your goals every day without leaving any stones unturned.

Eat high protein meals

You might have noticed that many people in the fitness industry suggests that others eat high protein meals. There's a reason for that, and the reason is that protein is one of the best macro-nutrients if you're looking to burn fat and to live a healthier life. Let's get into the Science as to why protein is essential when following an autophagy type of protocol, the first thing that protein does is preserve your muscle.

When you have more muscle mass new body, you will burn fatter. Therefore it is essential to have more protein to prevent muscle loss. Another thing protein is good at is burning off fat, protein is the macronutrient, which requires the most calories to digest. Which is why we need more protein you will burn fatter, because it takes much energy to digest and power is calories and calories as fat.

Another great thing that protein does is that it will not raise your insulin levels; unlike carbohydrates, protein does not increase your insulin levels when you eat it. Which is why it is a great idea to have more protein in your diet because you will get the energy and it will not raise your insulin levels? If your goal is to lose weight, look a lot better, and live a healthy life. Then you need to have enough protein in your diet. Protein is the building block to your body, and it will build muscle it will burn fat and most importantly keep you healthy for the days to come. Make sure that you are getting enough protein in your diet.

Rest

We talked about diet and working out so far, and the truth is those are one of the most important things to consider when following autophagy or any diet for that matter. However, the most critical thing we tend to overlook is the rest. If you're not resting enough, then you will not see results are you looking for.

There needs to be a right balance between exercising and rest, which is what we will talk about in the section of the book. Ideally, you should be resting at least twice a week from your workouts, so you should work out no more than five times a week throughout the day, and that includes your cardio and weight training workouts. When you don't rest, your body will counter-react to the stimulus you are providing it with to put on muscle and lose fat. If you don't want that to happen, make sure you give yourself twice a week of rest. Another form of rest would be sleep.

You need to ensure that you are getting an ample amount of sleep throughout the days, this will also help you recover from your workouts, more importantly, it will help you produce the optimal amount of hormones what you need for healthy body function. Some people say that you need 8 to 10 hours of sleep, but the truth is you can survive with 6 to 8 hours of sleep. Just make sure that you're getting enough sleep, to recover your body from working out and the daily stress that you might have acquired. Overall rest is an essential part of your fitness and health goals, so the last thing you need to do is overlook it.

Meditation

Since autophagy requires you to be in starvation to a certain degree, make sure you start meditation as it will allow you to focus more on your diet and more specifically help you with fighting off hunger. There are also many other benefits which would come along when the following meditation. It will help you to manage stress, many people don't know this, but having a proper meditation protocol will help you with coping with your anxiety. Keep that in mind, once you start your meditation.

Chapter 4: Which eating protocol to follow

One of the most well-known methods which have been known to facilitate with autophagy is intermittent fasting. In this chapter, we will give you seven means of following intermittent fasting. That way, you have a better idea on which method to follow and which you shouldn't.

Seven ways to intermittent fast

Since intermittent fasting has come out, there have been several methods which are being popularized by many fitness experts and gurus. At first, it was the simple fasting strategy which was fast for 16 hours and eat for 8 hours. But since then, we have discovered multiple different ways of fasting which are being used for fat loss and overall well-being.

In today's chapter, we will be talking about the seven main intermittent fasting methods which are being used by most fitness professional and experts out there. One of the best things in regards to following intermittent fasting is the ability to have choices. When fasting you have so many ways to go about it that it makes it very user-friendly, as you will learn later on in this chapter. Truthfully if you are deciding to follow intermittent fasting, then you should have no excuse. Intermittent fasting works with you instead of against you unlike most diets out there.

There are many ways to go about fasting, and we will be talking about those in this chapter. Just remember, even though you might have found the right fasting cycle for your lifestyle needs that doesn't mean it will fit your goal. For instance, if your goal is to notice more health benefits from fast rather than weight loss, then there are some fast that works better when compared to other options. Be aware, even though all fasts will help you lose weight and live a healthier life, you still need to make sure that you are following the plan which is right for your needs.

The 12 hours fast

Fasting for 12 hours is one of the ways to get started with fasting. That is the easiest way to learn how fasting works and to figure out how your body reacts to it. As I previously mentioned before, women tend to find fasting a bit more difficult because of their reproductive systems. Which makes a 12-hour fast an excellent tool for women to find out how their body reacts, and to slowly start to control their hunger cravings?

The 12-hour fast is very simple to follow, and you will be fasting for half the day and eating for half the day. When I put it like that, it doesn't sound so bad, does it? Although a 12-hour fast is still considered a fast and you will see some benefits from it, it won't be as drastic as something like a 16 hour fast or anything along that line. The 12-hour fast works are great to get your body to prepare for longer fasting and to show you what fasting feels like, it is merely a beginner's tool.

Nonetheless, we highly recommend 12-hour fast for women who are just starting off intermittent fasting. The best way to go about 12 hours fast would be to eat from 8 a.m. till 8 p.m. and then from 8 p.m. to 8 am not eat anything at all, even though this might sound easy for some it will still catch up on you. We recommend you follow the 12-hour fast for four weeks or until you feel like you can fast for a more extended period of time. But, most of the time four weeks does the trick for beginners. Even though, studies are showing that 12-hour fast tends to be the perfect time for fasting as tested on rats.

It is still recommended that you fast for a little bit of more extended time, as from personal experience and speaking with other experts in the field of intermittent fasting they recommend ideal fast should be 16 to 20 hours. Regardless when you fast for 12 hours, you'll start to see benefits such as your insulin sensitivity going up your fat loss will kick up a notch, and you will notice more mental focus.

The 12 hour fast does everything right, which makes the 12 hours fast a jack of all trades but a master of none. It is recommended that you only follow this method for a short period to see some results and to get used to fasting; you can pick any time frame you want to fast during. As we previously mentioned before, you can eat from 8 am to 8 pm and not eat from 8 pm to 8 am the next day. The timings won't make a drastic difference in the type of results you will be getting from the 12 hours fast. As long as you pick a time that works for you, then you should be good.

16 Hour fast

This is the fasting method, which has been popularized to be intermittent fasting. Many people use this method to lose weight and to gain some muscle especially men. But the 16 hour fast has been used successfully by women as well; Martin Bekhan who popularized this method truly lives by it. He has noticed the better fat loss, better health, and more muscle mass by following this plan. Now if putting on muscle is not your goal, the 16 hour fast still has some things to consider.

Most people notice when they start 16 hours fast is the ability to lose body fat without counting any calories or eating any specific foods. Since 8-hour window becomes too short to overeat, followers of the 16/8 intermittent fasting method tend to see amazing results in the weight loss department. From my personal experience, I can say that 16 by 8 was one of the best ways to lose fat, very easy to follow and 16 hours of fasting is not so hard, overall the results were tremendous. On top of losing weight, I noticed that my skin started to look a lot better which was precisely what I was looking for.

 In one of the newer studies done on obese individuals, they noticed not only fat loss but also reduction and blood pressure. Which means 16/8 method is excellent for fat loss and lowering the risk of cardiovascular diseases and heart diseases, even though this study was taken part on obese people it is still great to have been backed up by science? Bumping up from 12 hours to 16 hours, you will not notice a big difference in insulin sensitivity and mental focus. But, you will see more benefits towards that cellular rejuvenation and better results in fat loss.

You will also notice more detox benefits from the 16 hours fast if compared to the 12 hour, which makes the 16-hour fast a lot more similar to the 12 hours fast. Think of the 16 hours fast as the full version of intermittent fasting whereas the 12 hour fast is the trial version, even though there is only 4-hour difference between the two it stills makes up for a drastic change.

Once you start fasting for 16 hours instead of 12, you will notice the better fat loss and more health benefits from it. Just like the 12 hours fast, you can follow whichever way you want to pursue this fasting; the timings can be based on your lifestyle. We recommend fasting from 10 pm to 2 pm and eat from 2 pm to 10 pm, but make sure to pick a time that works for you.

Fast for 2 days per week

This fasting method was popularized by Michael Mosley, who is a doctor and journalist. Since this method has no studies to prove its benefits, it is still a method used by many people. Even though this method does not have any solid study to back it up, benefits which are stated include better brain function, Reducing the risk of heart disease, stroke, cancer and improving cholesterol levels.

This method can get tough to follow for some people. However, it will put you in a twenty percent calorie deficit which is a great place to be in if your goal is to lose body fat. This could be an excellent way to lose excess body fat if you can handle it, on that note let's talk about this method and how it works.

Also known as the 5:2 method is where the person eats an average amount of calories throughout the week and restricts their calories to five hundred/six hundred calories a day for two days. The guideline suggests five hundred calories a day for women and six hundred calories for men on fasting days. The method recommends you have two meals divided into your calories for the day when fasting, which means two meals of two fifty calories for women and two meals of three hundred calories a day for men.

Your calories will not be completely cut out throughout those two days, so make sure you are drinking a ton of water and other no-calorie liquids in between your meals on fasting days. Now the best way that you can go about using this method of fasting would generally be eating thru Monday to Friday then fasting over the weekend, and my recommendation would be fast when you don't have work or if you are doing anything physically demanding like working out.

This will ensure you don't feel tired or worst go hypoglycemic as you will be "fasting" for quite a long time, so make sure you are fasting on days you are not working or doing anything physically demanding. Also, the great thing about this method is that there is no food restriction during non-fasting days, which is definitely a good thing for some you foodies out there. Now there are some benefits to these methods, and let's talk about that.

 The primary benefit is that you will lose body fat and that too quite quickly, as a result of eating so little during those two days of fasting. I have personally followed this plan just as an experiment and I have to say, and I did lose body fat in those two weeks which I followed it. If your goal is fat loss without restricting your diet as much, then this method can be the one for you.

Another benefit claimed are lower cholesterol, lower risk of heart disease and cancer, which is fantastic for everyone following this method of fasting. But then again these benefits are claimed, not proven so don't follow this method if your goal is to lower the risk of diseases there are other fasting methods in this book that you can follow to get those benefits. The great thing about this fasting method is that you will get to eat what you want to eat, no need to restrict yourself on non-fasting days but if I were you, I would still be careful. Not to overeat if your goal is to lose body fat, so those are the benefits now let's talk about the cons.

This method is not ideal by any means, there are some flaws to this methods, and one of them was used in a positive but it is being used in con. In this method, you can eat whatever you want to eat, which is a flaw since people will eat a lot of junk food as an excuse and not do any justice to their health. I believe that fasting should be accompanied with a well-balanced healthy diet and having junk food on occasion, so I personally don't like the fact of having whatever you want on your non-fasting days as it can take away from the benefits of fasting.

Another flaw of this method is that it can be tough for some people to make it a lifestyle as fasting for two days straight can be a problem, but if it works for you then go for it. The main flaw is that there so no backing up the claims that this method is claiming. Although this is a fasting method and fasting has a lot of benefits which have been backed up, this method doesn't so as I said before don't follow this diet if your sole purpose is to lower the risk of diseases. If you follow a workout plan that requires strength training, then this fasting method might not be the one for you, as this method can hinder your workout quality as it did for some people.

So now you know all about the 5:2 method, this method can be used with great success if your goal is to lose body fat, and have basically no restrictions to your diet on non -fasting days. But please use this method for the right reasons; don't use it if you want a lowered risk of diseases as studies have not proved it.

Other fasting methods can be followed if your goal is lower the risks, and if your goal is to get stronger and put on some muscle then this method won't be ideal as this method can affect your workouts. All in all, if this method is being used for the right reasons, then it can lead you into great success in weight loss goals. If this method matches your lifestyle and goals, then follow this fasting protocol. But our recommendation would be to use this plan with a grain of salt and to only use for a short period. As we don't think this method is a sustainable fasting protocol like the 16/8.

Alternate day fasting

Very similar to the two days a week fasting, this method requires you usually eat on one day and the next day fast. For the fasting period, you are allowed to have 500 calories a day for women and 600 calories for men. However, you can take it up a notch and not eat any calories at all, which is not recommended by most but done by some. The whole reason behind the alternative fasting was to help people lose weight quickly; people have seen similar results as the 5:2 method where they lose a lot of body fat fast. This method has also been shown to lower the risk of diabetes, which is a great plus for people looking to lose weight and to lowers the risk of diabetes.

This method normally allows you to fast three days in a week, putting you at a 25% caloric deficit. Which is a little bit more than the 5:2 method, what I like about this fasting method is the frequency? If compared to the 5:2 method, you are fasting more frequently and more regularly. Whereas in the 5:2 method you are eating whatever you want for five days, and then fasting for two whole days straight, this makes it a little bit more reputable for me.

That being said, the same cons follow for this one. On your fasting days, you aren't genuinely fasting, and you can if you decide to but it not healthy especially for women to fast for 24 hours so frequently. Another disadvantage of this diet would be the allowance of eating whatever they want, although it is excellent for people who like to eat junk food it is not so healthy especially on fasting days. Most people will eat something non-dense like a slice of pizza, whereas you should be eating more of a dense meal to see better health changes overall.

Which makes this diet an excellent tool for weight loss, since it will help keep in a caloric deficit throughout the week. However, this diet is not a great way to see some health benefits from, making it very similar to the 5:2 fasting method. One great thing about this method when compared to the 5:2 method is the ability to maintain strength during workouts.

Since your fast will be very cyclical, your chances of losing a lot of strength will be lower which makes this diet ideal for someone looking to lose fat and maintain a healthy strength level thru-out.

 Finally, make sure that if you decide to follow this fasting protocol, it is for the right reasons. If you want to lose weight quickly and you have a comfortable going lifestyle, then this plan might be the answer for you. Also, just like the 5:2 method I would not recommend you follow this fasting method for a prolonged period of time as it can be unhealthy. However, besides all the negatives of this fasting protocol, there are a ton of positives especially if you are looking to lose weight.

Weekly 24 hour fast

The 24 hour fast has been used widely by many fitness professionals out there. Brad Pilon, the author of eat stop eat once, said: "prolonged calories restriction is the only way to fat loss." Which is the reason why the weekly 24 hours fast was created, easy as it sounds once a week you eat no calories. After you have completed the fast, eat regularly as you would if you were not fasting.

The whole premises behind this fasting protocol is to put you in a caloric deficit. For example, if you require 2,500 calories to maintain your weight then eat 2,500 calories a day but fast for one of those days. The claims of the weekly fasting method are, weight loss lowered the risk of diseases such as diabetes and many others. Unfortunately, in the weekly 24 hours fasts, the claims haven't been backed up with science. However, this fasting protocol has shown to speed up weight loss.

Many followers of this fasting protocol have seen fantastic weight loss effects. Which makes this a tremendous tool for fat loss, also really good for detoxing your body. The 24-hour fast will help you get rid of any toxins in your intestines and other organs, believe it or not digesting food is a hard task for our body. Not giving your intestines and other organs a break from digesting can lead to poor digestion, this is where the weekly 24-hour fasting shines. People who follow this fast, have noticed better digestion and healthier hair and skin because of cell rejuvenation effects it has.

The weekly 24 hours fast has shown to help with cell rejuvenation or also known as autophagy, which makes this protocol great for followers looking to lose weight and see results like better digestion and cell rejuvenation. Even though this protocol comes with a host of benefits, there are still some concerns.

Even though you are fasting for only one day a week, 24 hours fast can become very hard for some especially women because of the hunger craving.

It would be best if you had a great support system to pull through the 24 hours fast, another fall back of this fast would be the post-binge eating cravings. Many followers have noticed insane amounts of food craving the day after fasting if you over-eat throughout the week and fast for only one day, the chances of you losing weight will be slim to none. Make sure you have the will power to avoid these food cravings once you get them, as indulging in them would not be great if you are looking to lose body fat.

In conclusion, this protocol is ideal for people who have fasted for an extended period of time before. We would not recommend this fasting protocol to an absolute beginner, as it can be tough to follow through. Fasting has no benefit if you can't follow thru so make sure you pick the right one.

Meal skipping

This method is something people used to their body prepared for fasting, now to be clear I don't consider this to be as beneficial as most fasting protocol, and I repeat I don't believe this method to be as helpful as most fasting protocol. Now saying that would I recommend this method to someone else? The answer is yes! Why you ask, the simple reason this method is one of the easiest to follow, and it prepares you for fasting methods that will help you with better physical health and wellness. Would I recommend someone make this method their lifestyle, and the answer would be no?

Only consider this if you have never followed a fasting method before and you want to slowly build up to a longer fast which would make this method the one for you. Some readers can completely ignore this method and just start with other fasting method's listed above, if you have experience fasting before for a span of fifteen days then you should be able to follow a more "intense" protocols. None the less, let's talk about this method. The whole point of this method is for you to start skipping meals, in between the day to ease you into a longer fast.

So what you can do if you decide to follow this plan is to start by skipping breakfast then have some lunch and dinner, slowly building up to a longer fast. If you want you can even have a snack instead of skipping breakfast which will make it easier for you. The whole point is to make you feel comfortable before taking the big step, and this method allows you to take baby steps into the big realm of fasting. Which I think is the plus of this fasting method.

There are some benefits to this type of fasting method, one of the things that you might notice especially starting off is that you will most likely lose some fat. Often we don't realize how much we overeat, and the average person tends to eat more than he or she should. Most North American diet consists of foods which are loaded with carbohydrates, sugar and a ton of "bad fat" such as trans-fat in their diet. Which leads to most of the obesity issues in our society, one meal on average tends to be six hundred to a thousand calories per meal.

Now if you skip one meal every day for a week, you are looking to cut about forty two-hundred to seven thousand calories a week, a pound of fat has thirty five-hundred calories so you can defiantly see some fat loss benefits. This method will also give your gut a break from digesting all this processed food that some readers might be eating, which means better gut health overall. You can surely see all the benefits of this method, but this fasting method is something that you should not use as a protocol to lose fat in the long term as it can leave you malnour-ished in the end.

See our primary goal with this book is to show you how to live a healthy life both physically and mentally, sometimes our body gives us signals to skip meals and without even knowing you would skip a meal just because you felt like it. We are always using this method, but then the next day instead of three we have four meals and not to mention a big and unhealthy one. So our body always makes us clean our gut time to time organically, one thing people can get carried away within this method is since they skip a meal they think they can have anything their heart desires.

Which should not be the case, in my opinion, you need to be eating healthy doesn't matter if you choose to fast or not if you want to be free of health complications in future and looking good. By eating healthy we make sure to get all our micronutrients in, like our vitamins and minerals for the day and your macronutrients like your calories, fats, carbs and protein depending on your fitness and aesthetic goals.

Another thing that should not be left out is the consumption of water if you can't seem to skip the meal and you tend to get hungry, drink more water during your fast. Not only will that hydrate you, but it will also get rid of toxins in your body and help you with fat loss if that's your goal. At the end of the day, if you want to ease into this fasting lifestyle, you should use this method as a tool to get you up to a longer fast, so you don't fall off track. Just make sure you are using it for the right reasons if 12 hours fast is too much for you to begin with, then consider this protocol and move up from there.

The warrior diet

This method is more based on our ancestors eating habits, created by Ori Hofmekler this method suggest us to "eat like a warrior." In the earlier times fasting thru out the day and only having a four-hour window to eat a big meal was a norm for us humans, as Hofmekler thinks human were created to eat like this. This method was based on his belief system and how humans should be eating instead of using science-based evidence and studies. In this method you are allowed to have mostly whatever you want in that four-hour eating window, go by what you feel and also don't go by macronutrient count eat how much ever you want to eat.

Another thing which is advocated in this method is that you will be more suited for burning fat for energy, claimed by Ori Hofmekler. If you follow this diet, you will lose body fat and won't have to count calories. So in this method, you have to fast for twenty hours and have an eating window of only four hours.

Now if you are currently using the "16/8" method then switching up to the warrior diet won't be such a shock to your body, but if you are going to go from an average eating habit to this, then I will be hard for you physically. I would recommend starting with fasting for twelve hours and slowly building up to the twenty-hour mark. If fasting for twelve hours can get challenging for you, then I would suggest slowly skipping meals like breakfast, and then when that feels easy slowly skipping breakfast and lunch until you get to the point where you can fast for twenty hours of the day.

Now, the way its recommend to follow this method is to fast in the day time and eat at the night time, as warriors would do after hunting and preparing their meals at the end of the day. You can have your meals at any time even before going to bed, and this diet should be followed just like the ancient times like the warrior did, meaning fast in the morning and feast at night. In this diet, you can have fruits and vegetables but it's recommended you stay away from canned fruits and vegetables, also their juices.

In this method it's highly recommended to workout in an empty stomach, to stimulate a warrior lifestyle. It is suggested to work out for thirty to forty-five minutes of intense workouts, with the use of compound movements like pull-ups, push-ups, and squats which use more than one muscle group. You can still consume water, and other non-calorie drinks so don't be scared to workout not hydrated.

So in conclusion, this diet is based on a lifestyle which warriors had back in ancient times, which was a selling factor for some people including me. Since this diet has no science or studies to back it up, it can be a turn off to some people when it comes to following a fasting protocol. Since they might want to see health benefits like lowering the risk of diabetes and other things of that nature.

Even though this method is quite similar to "16/8", I think it should help lower risk of diseases but then again no research on it. On the other hand, if your goal is to feel and look like a warrior, this method will be the right one for you. Although I haven't followed this plan long enough to see drastic physical changes, I have met people who have completely transformed their physical appearance and health also their energy levels have drastically changed for the better. This method has re-sulted in success for most people, and when I followed it for one week, I felt like "16-8" is ideal for me as I was feeling the same on this method.

One thing I didn't like about this method is that you have to work out on an empty stomach, as with "16/8" I would workout fed. So if you don't mind working out on an empty stomach and you want to live a warrior lifestyle, then this method might be for you.

Even though this goes with no saying, always get recommended by your doctor before you follow this method or another method listed in this book. This method can be pretty hard for you in the beginning, make sure you don't go into it without easing into fasting. I hope you see the results that you are looking for following this fasting method.

We have now gone thru all the fasting methods, and you might have learned a lot from this chapter. Many people might say that fasting works differently on men as compared to women, but besides the hunger portion, it is the same. As long as you follow these fasts safety and with the guidance of your doctor, you should be fine.

Also if you read these chapters carefully, you might have noticed that some fasts are suited better for specific results. Even though all fasts will help you achieve fat loss and overall health benefits, there are some protocols tailored for weight loss and others which are suited for whole healthy well-being.

When you are picking out which fasting protocol to follow, consider lifestyle, and your goals as most of them will fit your needs. Overall know what you want out of intermittent fasting. Also, if you pick the right fasting protocol, then you should see the benefits which you have been looking to get.

Chapter 5: How to pick a plan with intermittent fasting

Now that you're aware of most of the intermittent fasting, we will now help you finalize on what plan you're going to be following when fasting. This chapter will help you realize what works for you when it comes to intermittent fasting because for someone 16/8 method might be better suited for some when compared to the 5:2 method. After this chapter, you should be fully equipped to start fasting. Later on in this book, we will talk about more intermittent fasting related stuff but for now, let us find out which plan to get started with when it comes to intermittent fasting.

Pick a plan

It is important that you pick the right fasting protocols for your needs, a couple of chapters ago we talked about all the methods of intermittent fasting. As you could tell, they were all different but none the less effective in their manner. Every fasting method tends to yield different types of results, so it is essential that you picked the right one which works with your lifestyle and your goals. What we will do is go through all the fasting method step by step and explain to you which one is suited for what type of goals and lifestyle, and after reading those you can decide on which one to start following. If that sounds good let's get started, we will start by talking about the 12 hours fast.

12 hour fast: As we previously mentioned, 12 hours fast is for someone who is a beginner in the realm of intermittent fasting. It is best followed by people who are just trying to get their feet wet, the 12-hour fast works many different ways. The 12-hour fast will help you clean out your digestive system, and will also help with weight loss. This fasting protocol is very similar to the 16 hours fast, and sometimes known as the baby 16 hours fast because it is a stepping stone to other fasting methods. If your primary goal is to lose fat, and to see some significant benefits from fasting, then this would be ideal for you. This fast is very manageable in regards to setting time for eating and fasting window, and you can fit in this intermittent fasting method at any time there is no specific window, which makes this ideal for busybodies.

16 hour fast: Very similar to the 12-hour fast, the 16 hour fast is one of the very popular fasting methods used by many. This method is for people who are trying to lose weight, build muscle and live an overall healthy life. If your goal is to get results from autophagy, then this fasting method might be for you, as this is one of the fasting protocols which have been proven to promote autophagy. This plan is ideal for people who are following the 12-hour fast and are looking for a bump, similar effects of the 12-hour fast it is just prolonged for 4 hours. If you're someone looking to get the most of the health benefits from intermittent fasting, then this plan is for you. Moreover, if you are someone who demands flexibility with the eating windows, then this plan would be better suited for you.

Fast for 2 days per week: Also known as the 5:2 method, this is one of the more intense fasting protocols. Even though there have been no studies showing the health benefits by following a 5:2 method, it is best known for drastic weight loss. If you're looking to lose weight quickly and efficiently oh, and this plan might be the answer for you. One thing to remember this plan whose better suited for women who had some experience with intermittent fasting, don't start following this plan if you're a complete beginner. This plan can be very easy to cope with on day to day basis, as you can merely fast when you are not working. Overall this plan is excellent for intermediate fasters who are looking to lose weight quickly, and one suggestion would be to not follow this plan for longer than four weeks.

Alternative day fasting: very similar to the 5:2 method, you fast for one day, and you usually eat the next day so on and so forth. Most of the time it works out be 3 days of fasting and 4 days off eating healthy. This method is a little bit more aggressive when it comes to weight loss, where the 5:2 method puts you in a 20% calorie deficit for the whole week this puts you in 25% calorie deficit making it an advanced protocol. If you are someone who is experienced with intermittent fasting and are looking to lose weight quickly, then I would highly recommend this plan to you, as this is one of the most aggressive yet safe ways to lose body fat. However, again make sure you follow it for less than 4 weeks.

Weekly 24 hour fast: It requires you to only fast once a week for 24 hours, quite frankly I'm not a fan of this fasting method, but I know many people use it. Some benefits are showing that it might help with cleaning out your gut, and helping you with overall weight loss as it will put you in 5% caloric deficit for the week. This plan can be used by anyone, as you can fast on the days off. Overall I am not a fan of this fasting protocol, but it is there for you to follow.

Meal skipping: Meal skipping is one of the most natural fasting protocols out there, if you are a complete beginner who is very scared to start intermittent fasting then this might be the stepping stone for you. Even though there will be minimal benefits from this fasting protocols, it will teach beginners to listen to their body. Overall helping you understand how your body works when in starvation mode, and help you show how to deal with hunger.

The warrior diet: The warrior diet, where you fast for 20 hours and eat for 4 hours. In the four hours you are allowed to eat whatever you want, just like any fasting method. Ideally, this fasting method was made for people looking to lose weight and gain muscle, hence the name. However, this diet is no different from the 16 hours fast, and there are no added benefits to fasting for extra hours from 16 to 20. If you are someone looking to make you're fasting a bit more challenging or shorten you're eating window in order to lower your caloric intake, then this plan can be for you. This plan can tire you out very quickly, from personal experience if you have a lot going with your work-life then stick with the 16 hours fast.

This information should help you tremendously with picking out the fasting protocol for your needs, make sure it is sustainable for you.

Take a look at your diet

Intermittent fasting works excellent, but it works a lot better when you eat healthier overall. For you to achieve better results from intermittent fasting, it needs to be health-focused meals.

You see when you start following intermittent fasting alongside a healthy diet, and magic starts to happen. What we will do is give you some pointers on how to begin observing intermittent fasting the right way.

We previously method before the macros and the eating patterns we recommended for people intermittent fasting, so let us recap them. If your goal is to lose body fat your macros should be 40% protein 20% carbs and 40% fats, whereas if your goal is to maintain your weight and reap the benefits of intermittent fasting, then we recommend following a macro protocol of 30% protein 40% carbs and 30% fats. If you want to lose weight, then you need to look at your diet making sure you don't go over your calories and macros. If you aren't eating healthy meals throughout the day, then you can slowly start to incorporate better meals.

Start by having one healthy meal when you break your fast and one meal of whatever you desire, and once you become more comfortable, you can make it two meals. Making you slowly start eating healthier, which will yield even better results overall. Yes, many people do get away with eating foods that aren't healthy, and yes, they see amazing changes. However, if you want to see over the top changes, then we recommend eating a bit more robust. Now there is no specific diet you need to follow, merely make healthier choices as this should help. You need to take a look at your food which you are eating and makes changes where necessary. It will be hard in the beginning but, it will eventually become more natural.

Learn to listen to your body

It's imperative that you listen to your body when you're fasting, listening to your body will help you understand one-stop and will not stop. Intermittent fasting for women can require extra attention, and that is why it is necessary to listen to your body. There are some telltale signs to look out for when doing intermittent fasting, know that most of the symptoms should subside within a week.

However, if they don't chances are you need to switch up your fasting protocol. One of the ways to tell the intermittent fasting is becoming way too hard for you, is when you start feeling cold chronically. Once you begin to feel cold chronically, that's a big sign that intermittent fasting is becoming very hard for you to follow if you feel cold throughout the day for three weeks plus then chances are it is time for you to lower the fasting intensity. Another sign to consider when you're intermittent fasting would be the extreme hunger.

The first couple of weeks you will feel extreme hunger, but if that keeps happening for over three weeks chances are your body is telling you that you can't follow intermittent fasting at this level. These are the significant signs you need to listen to your body when intermittent fasting, but always make sure you get your blood work done and get the professional help if you feel like intermittent fasting is affecting you physically. Best rules to live by when intermittent fasting if it doesn't feel right three weeks into it then stop. Nonetheless, symptoms could occur anytime, just be in-tuned with your body and make sure you are listening to it.

Helpful tips dealing with hunger

When following an intermittent fasting routine, it is crucial that you make sure that your appetite is under control to make sure fast isn't broken prematurely. Time and time again, many followers of the intermittent fasting have broken the fast prematurely just because they couldn't control their hunger. We will go multiple ways to deal with hunger, and overall help you continue with intermittent fasting. The first tip is pretty obvious, and that is to drink more water. Much of the time, hunger is thirst.

Meaning you will be able to control your eating desires by drinking more water, having more water through the day helps you tremendously to control your hunger. Another method for managing your hunger would be to drink more coffee and green tea, and caffeine has shown to suppress hunger which overall helps you with fasting. Just make sure the coffee or tea you drink does not contain any sugar or milk, as that could break your fast. Getting yourself busy will help you control your hunger, most of the time when we occupy ourselves with work we tend to forget the food.

Perhaps do some work, or household chores to keep yourself busy when you feel like eating. You can also exercise or go for a walk, and this will kill two birds with one stone. When you start walking, you will take your mind of fasting, and you will also burn some fat while doing so. If you are feeling more energetic, then you can go ahead and get a full workout. However, remember that you might feel hungry after the workout if you have no experience in managing your hunger. Now, if you are looking for a more relaxed way of managing your hunger, then we would recommend meditation.

Meditation works well when it comes to controlling your hunger, and it will also help you manage your mental stress if you have any. Make sure you are using this tool, to manage your hunger, and who knows you might really enjoy meditation. The final technique we recommend would be to eat more fibrous foods before you start your fast, as this will help you stay fuller for a long period of time. Many followers of intermittent fasting will eat junk food, this will actually make them crave foods faster than someone who ate a good healthy meal with a ton of fiber in it.

If you want to have a better less hungry fasting window, then we highly recommend you eat healthy meals with a ton of fiber in them before you start fasting. These are all the tips and tricks to dealing with hunger, make sure that you are following all these tips to control your hunger when fasting. Especially if it is your first three weeks fasting, as that is when you will notice most of the hunger cravings. These tips will help you tremendously to power through those first three weeks, and help you with completing your fast.

Track your progress

If you want to be successful with intermittent fasting, then you need to start tracking your progress. Tracking your progress is the main reason why most people continue on with intermittent fasting and why most people don't, and there's a reason for that. You see, when you start tracking your daily progress, you will begin to notice better results which will help you hold yourself accountable to it. There are three ways to track your progress when intermittent fasting, and we will talk about those today. The first way you can track your progress is by daily journaling, write down everything how you felt and how your body was feeling when fasting.

Not only will this teach you how to listen to your body, but it would also show your progress so if you're ever feeling down you can just go back and read past experiences and results with intermittent fasting and see how much better you have gotten. Another method to track your fasting would be to schedule out your whole week in terms of time frame like when it comes to fasting and eating window. Most people just go day-by-day fasting whenever they feel, which is fine but you'll see much better results if you figure out your whole week, so set up your fasting windows and eating windows.

This method would also help you stay accountable for your fasting goals. The third way to track your progress would be to measure your body composition every week. This will not only keep you motivated in terms of keeping you moving forward, but it would also help you see how you're progressing, and if changes are needed to be made. These are the three main ways to track your progress and to stay on track with intermittent fasting, and we recommend using all three.

Remember that most people give up or quit because they don't have a plan or a strategy to get somewhere. Once you start tracking your progress and tracking your intermittent fasting schedules, you will notice that you are a lot more accountable with your goals and you will begin to see better results.

We highly recommend you start tracking your progress and especially use these tools that we just talked about. There are also apps, which can be used to track your progress. If you don't like writing stuff out, then you can download apps which will help you to track your progress. Overall there should be no excuse not to track your progress. Also, we recommend you journal your body composition weekly and your journaling daily.

The journaling works a lot better when written daily since your emotions are at its peak when you write them out. However, if you feel that daily journaling can become hard, you can also journal weekly. Nonetheless, daily journaling is a lot better. Follow whatever feels best for you, but remember to track all three progress to see better results, doesn't matter how you track it as long you track it.

Chapter 6: Autophagy and Ketogenic

The minute we talk about switching to a diet, the first thing that comes to our mind is giving up on desserts. If you are someone, like me, who cannot resist a tasty dessert, then getting on a diet and staying put without cheating may get a bit problematic. If you have faced this issue, then I have some good news for you. You can lose weight by eating too, and I am talking about desserts as well.

The Ketogenic diet is the answer to all your diet-related prayers. While on this diet, you get to eat a wide variety of foods, fatty food included, and you are not required to stay off of desserts.

The Ketogenic diet works on a simple principle – eat fat to lose weight and stay away from the carbs. To be specific, the Ketogenic diet requires you to consume fewer carbohydrates, and turn to healthy fats as a source of energy. You need to keep the carb consumption below 100 grams a day. This implies that you will have to adapt to this new diet to stay healthy and fit. You are allowed to consume any quantity of protein or fat, depending on your weight-loss aims.

Every standard diet requires you to consume a proper mix of proteins, carbohydrates, and fats. However, as the Ketogenic diet needs you to control the number of carbs you consume drastically. Thus, you are depleting the reserves that your body has for energy. Therefore, your body will look for different ways to provide you with energy. One alternative way to get the power to burn is by using the fat that is stored in your body. Your body will begin to use this fat to fuel your body with energy.

However, not all organs can use these fatty acids for energy; they instead depend on the ketone bodies released by the liver for energy. When you reduce the consumption of carbohydrates, your body ends up producing more ketone bodies, which flow to your bloodstream leading to ketosis. Ketosis is nothing but a metabolic state of your body. At this stage, there is a decrease in production, and thereby, the utilization of glucose. When your body undergoes ketosis, your body will rely on using the fat reserves to provide you with energy.

That is how the Ketogenic diet works. As long as you eat Keto compliant ingredients, there is no stopping you from eating any variety of food, whether it is fried snacks or indulgent desserts

This should give you a basic overview of the Ketogenic diet. It is always better to do a Ketogenic diet if your goals to achieve autophagy. However, the Ketogenic diet can work when it comes to making total cell rejuvenation benefits. The way it works is pi helping you lower the carbohydrates. As we told you previously your body will first I just all the food and then proceeded to rejuvenate yourself. Even if you're not failing the Ketogenic diet, your body is doing it add a smaller scale. However, once you cut out all the carbohydrates from your diet, you will notice that your body will be a lot more efficient when it comes to achieving autophagy. More specifically, you will see that once you start following a Ketogenic diet, you will get into ketosis, which is very similar to autophagy. Many people call autophagy and Ketogenic diet or ketosis to be cousins. The reason why the column cousins are because they work at the same level.

Burns fat for fuel

You will burn a lot more calories following a Ketogenic diet than you would following any food out there. Most foods out there, make you eat 5 to 6 times a day every 2 to 3 hours. The reason why it won't work is that your glycogen will always be full and therefore your body will be using glycogen for energy and not be using its fat store. Here's the thing your body needs to be in the starvation mode to use fat stores, but your body is brilliant; it will not use body fat stores if it does not need to.

What Ketogenic diet does as I said is put you into starvation mode, once you're in starvation mode your body will use the fat for energy. Once your body starts using fat for energy, it will burn off the fat stores that you have giving you a more aesthetically pleasing physique. The reason why your body will be using the fat stored glycogen is because you will not be providing your body glycogen for a long time, when you don't give your body glycogen for a long period of time the only way it will function properly is to use the fat stores that you have in your body.

Another reason why a Ketogenic diet helps you burn more fat is that a puts you into ketosis. This is when your body will strictly use fat for energy and not glycogen. In later chapters, we will talk about how specific diets can help you burn fatter while following a Ketogenic diet. However, for now, know that the Ketogenic diet will help you burn fatter than glycogen throughout the day.

Boost your energy

Remember how we said Ketogenic diet boost your adrenaline, which is one of the reasons why you will have more power during the Ketogenic diet. When you have high amounts of adrenaline and your body, you will have more energy to do physical and mental tasks. Another way the Ketogenic diet helps you boost your energy is by not giving you any ups and downs in your insulin level.

Have you ever had the feeling of overeating food and feeling very tired right after, the reason why I feel exhausted right after is that your insulin is spiking up to digest their meal. When your insulin spikes up, you'll feel lethargy and tiredness. When Ketogenic diet, you will have no insulin spikes during your fast, which will allow you to have a sustained amount of energy throughout the day and therefore boosting power. These two things in combination will help your energy tremendously during a Ketogenic diet. Which is why the Ketogenic diet raises your energy, and when you mix it up with working out, then you are set on the part of excellent energy level throughout the day.

Before you get started

Before you get started, there are a couple of things to understand about the Ketogenic diet. The first thing is going to be making sure that the Ketogenic diet is followed the right way, as described in this book. If you don't do it right, then chances of you achieving your goals will go down significantly, so make sure you read this book very carefully before you start any fat Ketogenic diet protocol.

Consult a health physician

Before you start any diet, you need to consult with your position. As we talked about before how the Ketogenic diet cannot be suited for some people out there oh, so it is in your best interest to figure out if you are well enough to follow a Ketogenic diet. Ideally, you want to consult with someone, whom you can trust perhaps your doctor or a dietitian. However, whatever you do you make sure that you consult with a professional who knows what they're doing since we don't see what you look like or what your health complications are we can tell you if you're fit enough for Ketogenic diet or not. If you aren't fit enough for a Ketogenic diet, then perhaps try something new.

Keep it easy

Keeping it easy one of the best thing you can do to your body because the truth is it needs to feel less like a chore and more like a lifestyle so if you want to be successful in this, then it needs to feel comfortable. If you feel like a Ketogenic diet is a chore for you from the get-go, then the chances of you continuing with Ketogenic diet will go down drastically. Whatever you do, make sure the Ketogenic diet feels comfortable for you and that it is not a chore but more so of a lifestyle.

Now there's a couple of ways to keep it easy, and the first way would be to start slow. We have to explain to you how to start easy, so start with that and then move on to the big stuff. Overall you want to make Ketogenic diet and manageable natural part of your life, and you have to figure out how you're going to do that. We can give you some pointers and some tricks on how to do that, but it is for you to find out what works for you and what doesn't.

Keep it simple

Please don't make things harder than they're supposed to be, especially when you're the Ketogenic diet. It is straightforward to make things hard when following a Ketogenic diet, as there many things to consider and many things to do. The best thing you can do is keep things simple; the way to keep things simple is by not overthinking stuff. By that I mean, not overthinking how much food you're missing while fasting or what kind of foods you will be eating when you break your fast. Just take it one step at a time, when you start taking one step at a time is a lot easier for you to continue with the Ketogenic diet and it won't feel like such a chore.

Also, when you try to keep things simple, you need to realize that it is in your best interest to stay away from external information which might throw you off. Such as new diet fads that are coming out, make sure you stay in your lane and follow a Ketogenic diet for the time being. Please stick to the plan, do not deviate from it, and finally, keep things simple.

Chapter 7: Things to avoid

As we recently talked about the benefits of eating healthy foods when autophagy, we will not talk about the diets you need to stay away from in order to achieve optimal success during autophagy. There are many diets which are supposedly healthy for you when they're not, and unlike autophagy, they're not sustainable for an extended period. Nonetheless, we will talk about the main things to consider while picking out your eating habits. Make sure you read this chapter very carefully to see optimal success.

Most diets are not maintainable

As you might know, how many foods aren't maintainable for an extended period, the simple reason behind it is that they make you do too much in a short period. Which is why we don't recommend following any diet when following autophagy, merely eat healthy and nutritious.

Although there is one diet, we think that goes well with autophagy. We will talk about that diet and detail later on in this book. Nonetheless, let's talk about the reasons why most diets are maintainable, the reason why they are maintainable, especially during autophagy because they make you under eat a lot. When you under-eat during autophagy, the chances of you giving up are incredibly high, don't get me wrong being in a caloric deficit while autophagy is fine, but to do it right is another thing.

There is a sweet spot, between autophagy and caloric deficit and if you mess that up, then chances of you maintaining a proper eating schedule will go drastically down. For now, merely eat healthy nutritious meals during autophagy. Later on, we will show you a diet which can help you lose even more body fat.

Fad diets can be harmful

You have probably seen these diets before, and they are very available in magazines. Stay away from fad diets as much as possible, and there's a reason why because they don't work at all and they will put you in a worse position health-wise. When you are in a caloric deficit for an extended period, it can mess with your hormones and fat loss will worsen in the long run, the worst thing is that affect your metabolism. When you don't eat enough calories for a sustained period, it will change your me-tabolism in the long run.

Another thing that fad diets can do is cause eating disorders. Many people don't know this, but eating disorders are one of the biggest things people face when they follow fad diets. Depending on the fat intake, it could be low carbs or no carbs, which are impossible, or sometimes surviving on liquid for the rest of your days. This is not ideal for anyone looking to lose weight, so the best thing you can do is stay away from these diets and focus on autophagy.

Yo-Yo diet

Similar to fad diet, yo-yo dieting is when you lose weight, and you gave back really fast. There have been many studies showing that you're worried that he was not optimal for many people, as it slows down your metabolism, which in the long term cause you to gain more weight. Trust me you don't want to do yo-yo diet in the long-term, let's talk about couple things that you might be doing which could be similar to yo-yo dieting, the first thing that you might be doing what you're somebody yo-yo dieting has too little carbs.

Your body needs a certain amount of carbs throughout the day to survive, and it to lose weight you need to give your body just the right amount of carbs to put it into a caloric deficit well not damaging the hormones and metabolism. If you feel incredibly sluggish throughout the day, and it has been going for an extended period, then you need to revisit your diet. Perhaps adding more carbs to nutrition, are just more calories in general throughout the day can cause you to get out of that cycle. Nonetheless, if you are on yo-yo diet get away from it, if you do not keep doing what you are doing, chances are you are in a much better place.

Eating disorders

If you are facing any eating disorders, Or if you don't know what eating disorder is. It is when you can't control what you're eating, or it is hard for you to eat healthy, to just put in layman's term. The best way to avoid and eating disorders is to stay away from yo-yo dieting and are any fad diets. The good thing about autophagy is that prevent you from getting into any eating disorders. As it teaches you how to control your appetite and when to eat it, which is very healthy for your body. If you think you're facing eating disorders, then talk to your doctor as they might be able to help you a lot better.

How diets can make you binge

So far we have talked about many reasons why many foods can put you in a very unhealthy place, especially cause you to binge.

The idea behind why you bench while on a diet, is because there are too many restrictions. You need to follow a diet where they are not a lot of restrictions on can help you sustain it for an extended period, the only reason why you binge while following a diet is that there are too many restrictions, if you want to avoid binging merely pick a plan which works for you.

A form of starvation

Most diets are a form of fasting, the reason why it's because you're not getting enough nutrients throughout the day. Most diets don't allow you to eat enough food, and therefore, your body goes into starvation mode. A certain amount of starvation mode is excellent, and the most have put you in a position where you don't have even enough nutrients to have a proper function body. Which is why dieting can become a form of starvation, so try and stay away from it as much as possible.

Diets can be restricting

As you know, diets have many restrictions, such certain foods you can't eat or calories you can consume. Which is why you mustn't follow a diet as it can cause you to become more proactive towards indulging in cravings, not only that there are some restrictions which don't make sense at all. Most diets suggest many "stupid" things such as not eating solid foods and surviving on liquids. Which is not a great idea if you are looking towards a healthy lifestyle overall, I can keep going on my restrictions which come along with diets, but you get the point. Stay away from foods until you have found the right one for you.

Increased craving when dieting

The difference between autophagy and dieting is this, and when you're autophagy, you start losing cravings for certain foods as compared to dieting when you do not lose any needs and say you gain more.

Many people notice a lot of cravings while dieting, mostly for sugars as this is what they're missing in their diet. If you see cravings for foods that have a lot of sugar and chances are you're not eating enough food. Moreover, yes you can still lose weight while eating the right amount of food, you have probably noticed Cravings before as I'm assuming you've tried out a diet here and there.

Which is why we recommend you stay away from dieting, as of right now we're just all the problems related to dieting to steer you off from it. Don't get me wrong, at the beginning of autophagy, and you will notice many cravings for food. However, if you give it a week or two, the Cravings will go away, and in fact, you will start to notice that you are in control of what you eat and when you eat.

Diets can cause weight gain

Remember how we talked about your metabolism slowing down when the following traditional type of dieting, well it is correct. When you die for an extended period, and you lose the right amount of weight, the chances are you will gain it back rather quickly. You see when you don't eat enough food, your metabolism will go down, and once your metabolism goes down, you will start to notice a tremendous amount of weight gain. Which is why guys recommend to cycle off at a time to time because they know that it's causing damage to your metabolism? Meaning, if you don't want to gain weight, then don't diet as you will gain it back very quickly.

Your diet might have been successful, but chances are you will gain the weight back
As we explain to you how you will increase your pressure again while dieting, it is widespread to see drastic weight loss. It is merely because you will be in a caloric deficit, which will put your body in starvation mode. However, once you get out of the starvation mode, your body will go into hibernation mode.

This is when you will store all the fat that you have for energy. Anything you eat will be used in moderation for power, putting most of it into your fat stores. Which makes sense because your body doesn't know when it will get food again, so make sure you are aware of the fact that you will gain the weight back. If you happen to be successful dieting, and you're noticing that you're gaining your weight back. Then the only way you can fix it is by the following autophagy because autophagy not only raises your metabolism, but it keeps your body in a healthy level of starvation mode. This will make your body lose fat, and maintain a healthy metabolism rate, so you don't gain your weight back ever again.

Cholesterol norepinephrine and epinephrine increase

These hormones are one of the essential hormones in your body, as they ensure that you lose weight at a specific rate. When you're dieting chances, your norepinephrine and epinephrine will increase, which is good for weight loss. However, you don't want unhealthy spikes of these hormones, as something that comes up quickly will shoot down so rapidly be aware of the fact that when you're dieting extremely, it will go up but once you stop it will shoot back down.

On the other hand, when autophagy you hormone levels will increase and stabilize at the top, causing no unnecessary side effects what you might expect from dieting. Just be aware that before you start any diets, and as always we recommend the following autophagy.

Your body may have a problem releasing waste

You have to realize that your body is brilliant when it finds out that it is in a starvation mode, it will hold on to everything possible for energy. Which also includes your waste, this will cause a big problem in your body if you can't release your waste correctly. There are two ways dieting affects your waist releasing, the first way is by your body holding onto your trash for energy and the second way is by your body not getting enough nutrients or fibers to digest the food properly and turn it into the garbage.

There are some ways to ensure that it doesn't happen, the first way would be to ensure that you're getting enough fiber in your diet if you want to make sure that you're getting rid of your waste correctly then make sure your fiber intake and do water intake is up there. Dieting or not, you need to make sure that fiber intake and water intake is at a healthy amount for you to get rid of your waste. Another way to ensure that your body doesn't hold on to garbage is effortless not to diet.

Lack of energy when working out

When you're not eating enough food, or I should say nutritionally dense food, then the chances of you having a great workout will drop down drastically. To ensure that you don't have bad workouts, start eating more food and more specifically healthy food. Has anyone died and you don't get enough nutrients in your body and therefore you will have a lot less energy when working out or hitting the gym.

The gym is also a big part when it comes to losing weight and staying healthy overall. Which is why we recommend you fuel your body? Accordingly, this would be to ensure that you have a great workout at the gym, and you get the most out of your workouts. Couple of ways to do that, as first make sure you're getting enough micronutrients such as vitamins and minerals. The second way to do that is to eat enough food, and once these two things are in place, you will healthily lose weight while ensuring that you don't lose your health.

When autophagy, you start to notice that your energy will become more abundant during your workouts, which is why it is a great idea to follow autophagy working out is a big part of your life. Nonetheless, the main takeaway from this would be that your diet doesn't negatively affect your workout.

Magic weight loss scammers

Finally, we need to talk about the big elephant in the room, which is the which are the magic weight loss scammers. You have seen them, and you already know what they are like. The best thing you need to do is to stay away from these weight loss scammers as they don't care about anything else but your money.

Couple ways to tell that they are magic weight loss scammers is if they make claims which are too good to be true, as you might have heard the saying "if it sounds too good to be true it is." If you have a feeling that these weight loss cameras might be genuine, then the first thing you need to do is ask you how professional or your doctor about the diet the scammers are offering.

If your doctor or your fitness expert doesn't agree with it, then chances are it is a big scam, like we always say do your research before you start anything, which is why we wrote This Book, to show you how autophagy works. However, for now, your goal is to stay away from fad diets, more specifically, weight loss cameras, which will do whatever it takes to get your money.

Chapter 8: How to make this a life-style

We will talk about what you should be doing, to make sure that you are not failing in your endeavors to start this diet to live a healthier life overall. This chapter will show you what you could be doing to make this diet your lifestyle and to not only help you to start the autophagy and stay on track but also to live with this eating plan for the rest of your life. These daily patterns will help you to not fail on your diet, and we understand that you might fail a couple of times in any diet, and it is understandable to do so. Nonetheless, this chapter will show you how to make sure you are consistent and not failing. These habits have been followed by many successful people, to get optimal results in all of their aspects of life, whether it be fitness related or anything else. Make sure you start implementing all of these habits after you are done reading this book as it will help you to make this diet your lifestyle. The reason why this chapter might sound philosophical is that the only way you will see success with this diet is if you do it consistently. For you to do that, you need to change your current lifestyle by being more productive and disciplined. You have to remember, healthy eating is more than just a meal; it's a lifestyle.

Plan your day ahead

Planning your day ahead of time is crucial, not only does planning out your day help you be more prepared for your day moving forward, but it will also help you to become more aware of the things you shouldn't be doing, hence wasting your time.

Moreover, planning your day will truly help you with making the most out of your time, that being said, we will talk about two things 1. Benefits of planning out your day 2. How to go about planning out your day. So, without further ado, let us dive into the benefits of planning out your day.

It will help you prioritize:

Yes, planning out your day will help you prioritize a lot of things in your day to day life. You can allow time limits to the things you want to work on the most to least, for example, if you're going to write your book and you are super serious about it. Then you need a specific time limit every day in which you work on a task wholeheartedly without any worries of other things until the time is up. Then you move on to the next job in line, so when you schedule out your whole day, and you give yourself time limits, then you can prioritize your entire day. The same thing goes for your diet, make sure you allocate time for prepping your meals for the next day, which will allow you to have meals ready for you when you need it hence making it easy for you to continue with your diet.

More focus on the task in hand:

This point is quite similar to the previous point, once you have started to plan out your day and you have become more aware of the things that you are about to do. With the time limit on all task that you do daily, it will create an urgency to get as much of the job done as you can before time is up and you are moving on to your next appointment. Which will help you be more focused on the task at hand and get more things done? Many people consider healthy eating to be time-consuming, which it isn't if you prioritize your time the right way. If you cook your meals the day before and you set times for your meal, then it should not be a problem.

Work-life balance:

You see, once you start planning out your whole day, you become more aware of your time and how to balance it out. Once you begin to write out your entire day ahead, you will know precisely what you are doing that day, so you don't have to do anything sporadically throughout the day. Always plan some time for yourself every day where you can wind down read a good book, meditate or maybe hang out with your friends and wind down. You will feel refreshed the next day, having to wind down and "chill out" will only make you a more productive person.

Planning out your whole day ahead will not only help you prioritize better. It will also help you be more focused on your task in hand and will help you have a better work-life balance. This also means that you are eating foods that you like once in a while; this will help you to stay motivated with the diet that you are following. So now that we have covered the benefits of planning out your day let's dive into the how to's when it comes to planning out your day.

Summarize your normal day:

Now, before we start getting into planning out your whole day ahead, you need to realize that to plan your entire day, you need to know precisely what you are doing that day. Which means you need to write down every single thing you do on a typical day and write down the time you start and end, it needs to be detailed in terms of how long does it take for your transportation to get to work, etc.

Now after you have figured out your whole day, you can decide how to prioritize your day moving on could be cutting out a task that you don't require or shortening your time for a job that doesn't need that much time. After you have your priorities for the day, you can add pleasurable tasks into your day like hanging out with your friends, etc.

Arrange your day:

You must arrange your day correctly, so the best way to organize your day is to make sure you get all your essential stuff done earlier in the day when your mind is fresh. After that's done, you can have some time for yourself to relax and do whatever it is that you want. But make sure you get all the things that need to be done before you can move on to free time for yourself. Another thing that will help you is to set time limits on each task, and once you start setting time limits, you will be more likely to get the job done.

Remove all the fluff:

So, what I mean by that is remove all the things that are holding you back from achieving your goals. Make sure you remove all of the things that are holding you back from getting the things that you need to be doing. If you have time for the fluff, do it if not, then work on your priorities first. In conclusion, planning out your day will help you tremendously! Make sure you plan out your day every day to ensure successful and accomplished days.

Be Grateful

We will be talking about how to be grateful and what are the benefits of being thankful for what you have! Now believe it or not being grateful every day will help you get more things done while keeping your mood elevated, see when you're thankful for the things you have you will start to feel like your mind will be in peace and joy. When your account is in order and comfort, you will be more productive with all the tasks ahead of you that day. Being in a grateful state of mind will help you become less stressed and more positive, which will help your work quality by ten folds. So, you must stay grateful not only for better work performance but to also be in a peaceful state of mind. This will also help you to do more positive things with your diet, such as eat clean through the day. Let's discuss the three main benefits of being thankful.

Helps you start your day:

Of course, if you start your day in a happy mood, you will more likely be keen to do more stuff and be more productive. If you read up on the most dedicated peoples and their day to day life, you will know that successful people tend to practice the same habits which I am going to be talking about in this chapter. The benefit of saying things you are grateful for, first thing in the morning will boost your positive vibes when you talk about the items, you're thankful for you will complain a lot less and attract negative vibes which is something we don't want! You always want to be in a positive mood as much as you can. To make sure you are in a positive vibe, write or say things you are grateful towards.

You will become more approachable:

Yes, being grateful will make you more approachable! Believe it or not, people do sense your "vibes" when you walk into the door. When you're more thankful about life, you are happier and more positive, which is what people want to be around. Who knows the next person you see could be an opportunity for you to grow your business or get a new job! So always make sure you are in a great mood and counting your blessings still, as good things will come to you.

Lowered stress levels:

I think this point is very self-explanatory, let me ask you this what most people are stressed about? Lack of resources plain and straightforward. A lack of resources creates 99% of the stress. Once you start counting what you have rather than what you don't have, you begin to become a lot less stressed, which is suitable for your physical and mental health! So, make sure you always stay in a grateful mood. If you want to learn more about how being grateful can change your life, I recommend reading "The Magic" by Rhonda Byrne.

So, all in all, being grateful will help you live a better life and be more successful. Now you might be wondering how to be thankful throughout the day since it is so hard to block out ungrateful thoughts, well I'll show you three techniques that will help you combat your ungrateful thoughts and keep you in a grateful "vibe" most of your life.

Write ten things you are grateful for every morning:

You see, writing what you are thankful for will make your life a lot easier and help you start your day in gratitude. What I would like you to do is first get a notebook/diary, then as soon as you wake up, I want you to write ten things you're grateful for. This could be anything from small as having water to drink to have a nice car, the whole point of this is to make you start your day in gratitude as the way you start your day is the way your entire day is going to be most of the time. So, make sure to start your day on the right foot by writing down ten things you're grateful towards.

Don't forget the 1:5 ratio:

This is something I came up with, and it works great for me, you see whenever I say something I am angry or not grateful for I always say five things I am super thankful for right after to get myself into the grateful "vibe" in the beginning this method will be your best friend as it will save you from killing your "vibe".

Cut out negative people:

This task might be the hardest to do, but it is quite essential, see the people who you are around are the people who will create your personality. So if you are around negative people, you will develop adverse circumstances for yourself, so if you are around people who are not upbeat about life and find everything wrong and never see the good in anyone, you need to cut them out and be around people who are happy and ready for what life has to offer. Now I get it, some cynical people can be your family members, and you can't cut them out, the best thing to do is 1. Make them understand what they are doing wrong 2. Show them how they can change their life. And if they still want to remain the same, then keep your distance.

In conclusion, you must be in a grateful "vibe" as it will not only help you with your mental and physical health, but it will also help you attract better people and better circumstances. Don't forget to practice the three methods we discussed in this chapter for you to be in a grateful 'vibe" throughout the day and life! That being said I hope this chapter shed some light on the importance of being grateful and how it can make or break your life, and I hope you don't take this chapter lightly being grateful is the most critical thing you can do to turn your life around. So be thankful!

Now that we have covered the part of being grateful, and how it can help you with your day to day life and eating habits. Let us give you some concrete ideas on how to change the way you live your experience and to make it better.

Stop multitasking

I think we are all guilty of this at a time, and if are multitasking right now, I need you to stop. Now multitasking could be a lot of things, it could be as small as cooking and texting at the same time, or it could be as big as working on two projects at the same time. Studies are showing how multitasking can reduce your quality of work, which something you don't want to do if your goal is to get the best result out of the thing that you are doing. That being said, there are a lot more reasons as to why you shouldn't be multitasking, so without further ado, lets dive into the primary reasons why multitasking can be harmful.

You're not as productive.

Believe it or not, you tend to be a lot less productive when you are multitasking. When you go from one project to another or anything else for that matter, you don't put all your effort into your work. You are always worried about the project that you will be moving into next. So, moving back and forth from one project to another will affect your productivity if you want to get the most out of your work you need to be focused on one thing at a time and make sure you get it done to the best of your abilities. Plus, you are more likely to make mistakes, which will not help you work at the best of your ability.

You become slower at your work.

When you are multitasking, chances are you will end up being slower at completing your projects. You would be in a better position if you were to focus on one project at a time instead of going back and forth, which of course helps you complete them faster. So, the thing that enables you to be faster at your projects when you're not multitasking is the mindset, and we often don't realize how much mindset comes into play. When you are going back and forth from one project to another, you are in a different mental state going into another project which takes time to build and break. So, by the time you have managed to get into the mindset of project A you are already moving into project B, it is always best that you devote your time and energy one project at a time if you want it to doe did an at a faster pace.

Affects your creativity.

This is a significant disadvantage of multitasking, and studies are showing that multitasking can negatively affect your creativity. When something requires too much focus from your end, it becomes harmful to your creativity, and you need a lot more attention when multitasking compared to working on one thing at a time. If you want to succeed and live a better life, then you need to be creative, so if multitasking affects your creativity, then you need to stop doing that.

By now, you can see how multitasking can hinder the ability for you to work at your best. These three things listed above are a no-no when it comes to living a better and more productive life; not only does multitasking help not be prolific but makes you slower and less creative. So, all the benefits you thought you were getting multitasking was not accurate after all, nonetheless, by now, you might be wondering how to go about working most efficiently. Well, the best way to put it is to work on one project at a time, I want you to put all your time and energy in the project you are doing currently and not worry about other projects. Make sure you set yourself goals when you start the project which will help you be more efficient and faster at your work, so an example would be "you will not move on to another project until project A has been completed" or you have managed to hit a certain threshold at that specific project. So, to sum it all up.

Do one project at a time

Don't move on until it is completed or you have managed to hit a certain threshold

Set yourself a goal (time, quality, etc.)

All in all, multitasking will do you no good. It will only make you slower at your work and make you less productive. Making sure you stop multitasking is essential, as it will only help you live a better life. One thing to remember from this chapter is to put all your energy at one thing at a time, and this will yield you a lot of better projects or anything that you are working towards to be great. If you want to be more successful and live a better life, you need to make sure your projects are quality as I can't stress this point enough. You are probably reading this book because you want to get better at living your life or achieve goals that you just haven't yet, one of the reasons why you are not living the life that you want or haven't reached your goal could be a lot of things but, one of the items could be the quality of your work which could be taking a hit because of you multitasking. So, review yourself, and find out why you haven't achieved your goal and why you are not living the life that you want.

Then if you happen to stumble upon multitasking being the limiting factor or the quality of your work, I want you to stop multitasking and start working on one project at a time while giving it your full attention. What you will notice is that your work will have a higher quality and will be completed in a quicker amount of time following the steps listed above, which will change your life and help you achieve your life goals in a better more efficient way.

After reading this chapter, many might be thinking that this is more of a self-help book than it is a diet book. The truth is that we want you to understand how to live a better life by changing the habits that you are currently following. Following a diet and making it a lifestyle is a lot more work than you think it is. For you to make it easy, you need to understand that you need to change your habits to be successful at this diet, which means you need to change the way you move the way you think and the way you perform. This chapter gives you a clear idea on how to start living a better life by changing up your habits, once you do change your practices you will notice that following autophagy diets as a whole will be straightforward for you.

The reason why it will be straightforward for you is that you will change the way you move and the change the way you live your life in general. Changing the way you live your life will not only help you get better results, but it will also help you to follow this diet as a lifestyle, many people confuse food as not being a part of a lifestyle, and it is something that they're supporting to better their health. But the truth is that when they're following a diet, they don't realize that it needs to be a lifestyle for it to be a health benefit, if you want to be healthier then you need to make sure that you're taking care of your health 24/7 365 days a year. Which means you need to make this a lifestyle, and for you to make this a lifestyle, we need to understand some self-help techniques to keep it sustained for a more extended period. Which is why this chapter is more self-help oriented, we wanted to make sure that this book is different than any other books that you've read when it comes to the following autophagy. The way we're going to be delivering it is by showing you how to change your lifestyle for the better instead of the worst. We're not just going to give you foods to eat and how to the following autophagy, but in fact, we're going to change the way you eat overall and to make it a better experience for you once you start getting into this diet. With that being said, I hope this chapter was helpful to you.

Conclusion

Thank you so much for downloading the book *autophagy: find out how fasting improves your health. An indispensable guide that helps you heal your body and lose weight with the self-cleaning autophagy system.* As you can tell, after reading this book, we went through a lot of things when it comes to autophagy and how to follow the right way to see the proper results.

Keep in mind that when it comes to this method, you have to make sure that your diet is perfect or at least good to see results. As you read this book, we talked about intermittent fasting and how can help you to see your results from autophagy. Also, a Ketogenic diet can help you tremendously with autophagy.

You are keeping that in mind, it is now in your hands to decide what kind of diet you're going to be following and how you're going to get there based on the knowledge provided to you in this book. What we did a great job in this book was to help it be more customized. More specifically, how to figure out how to pick out the right plan for your needs and how to achieve the true autophagy that you have been looking for. With that being said, we conclude this chapter thank you so much for reading it till the end, and we hope you enjoyed this book.